The Uncharted Natural Art

of

Conceiving, Pregnancy Prevention
and
Childbirth Spacing

Danny Saturday

Published by:
2DHouse Publishing
Monterey Park, California
626-221-1768
Email:2dhouse@earthlink.net
Website: www.2dhousepublishing.com

Distributed by:
Professional Publishing House
1425 W. Manchester Ave. Ste B
Los Angeles, California 90047
323-750-3592
Email: professionalpublishinghouse@yahoo.com
www.professionalpublishinghouse.com

Cover design: Jay De Vance, III
First printing January 2013
978-0-615-76647-8
Library of Congress Control Number: 2013932441
10987654321

DEDICATIONS

This book is dedicated to my late mother, Teodorica, a rural community midwife in the city of Candon, Ilocos Sur, Philippines.

My late wife, Milagros, a labor and delivery nurse for over 30 years.

My only daughter, Melanie, and my first granddaughter, Mia.

ACKNOWLEDGMENTS

I want to thank Duchine, my business partner for believing in my work and for all his encouragement and support.

Thanks to my dearest partner for life, Marissa Zari-Morfe for your support.

NOTE FROM THE AUTHOR

In order to understand the full spectrum regarding the uncharted natural art of conception, pregnancy prevention, and childbirth spacing, it's important that you can visualize information such as: How eggs develop, how sperm develops, and how sperm and the egg meet. Therefore, I have provided an appendix in the back of this book with illustrations that will help you to understand the process of ovulation and conception.

TABLE OF CONTENTS

PREFACE

⊂══⟨⟩⊢

This journal is long awaited. Over three decades, this idea brewed a persistent feeling of desire to write and share this method with everyone in need of guidelines, in classrooms or in the privacy of their own bedrooms around the world. This information is timeless: today and for the future. A key component to this notion is an open mind. Concepts elaborated here are not unfamiliar or new. However, this uncharted methods are the two models reconstructed in order to push us to think beyond tradition and discuss what is attainable through natural processes. The uncharted natural methods: (1) Controlled conceiving process (2) Pregnancy prevention use of the Absticulate Method for prevention and child spacing. Through this discussion, I hope to promote honesty, communication, and trust among couples, which are needed to maintain a positive state of mind preceding the process of these practices.

The information presented is for educational purposes for childless couples, mothers with multiple children, mature singles, as well as teens. It can provide an insight into natural alternatives for people hoping to seek different perspectives and/or complimentary actions towards conceiving or pre-venting a child. I was eager to disclose these thoughts, but I remained patient that life would steer and build us until the time was right. The intensity to share waned as I was preoccupied with my budding career and young family life. Nonetheless, I took every opportunity to engage in a friendly dialogue with my friends and family due to my desire to assist them and enlighten them about childbearing practices.

Preface

For many years, I helped married childless couples with this method. Some were skeptical and still choose not to believe it. Some thought that what I said was a joke. Often most told me "we don't need it" or "we've tried all kinds of things already," which included medical professional advice. Eventually, these people seeking professional help soon realize that time is running out on them. The point I hope to stir up is to merely consider the proposal to either compliment or precede current choices and options, because these natural processes require dedication and sincerity to humanity's sexual desire and sexuality.

This method may not work for everyone. It may seem unconventional to the norm; it pushes boundaries beyond the comfort level of an average conversation. However, for those who are looking for something different, alternative, or complimentary, they must commit to practice, while following this method. Soon individuals will soon discover that this technique may be a good alternative for childless couples who have difficulties conceiving and/or preventing to conceive.

Technology can take precedence over natural forms of conception for women who have experienced difficulties

13

in conceiving. Today, in vitro fertilization is the primary procedure used throughout the world to help distressed women, especially affluent married women, to conceive. This is the most expensive alternative form of conceiving. In addition, women facing financial hardship are often used as a surrogate to carry someone else's child. This procedure is known as petri-dish or test-tube babies.

An assortment of material regarding conceiving, pregnancy prevention, and childbirth spacing is posted all over the world-wide web, providing many women an opportunity to share their own experiences. Medical journals and research publications are also available and provide results and explanations about these matters, but are frequently difficult to comprehend by most people because of the technical and medical language employed. Most of all, the male perspective is commonly misunderstood, insignificant, and underestimated. Therefore, the respect of what both women and men contribute to the process is what makes these methods successful.

INTRODUCTION

INTRODUCTION

On an island at the far eastern part of the world stood a small stilt house made out of bamboo with neatly arranged, sun-dried coconut leaves. With the coastal reef set on the horizon, this poor fishing village was alive with inhabitants that lived off the sea and cultivated coconut trees. And on a little space of fertile land, they managed to grow vegetables and fruit trees for their own daily sustenance and barter.

Over the years they struggled. Eventually, this community became educated and their lifestyle changed gradually and then dramatically. Roads and electricity connected the neighborhoods. Automobiles, TVs, cable, computers, cell phones, then the internet and iPods, and modern kitchen appliances appeared. However, the natural beauty of this place remained untouched despite the modernization of the town and surrounding communities.

This place is being etched day by day but maintains its natural beauty. The salty sea wind blows through the canopy of trees, providing a fresh cool breeze throughout the village. Every day, the sunset provides a miraculous panoramic view of a painter's color pallet from pale pink to dark crimson, and from orange into deep royal purple. People are fascinated as they watch the celestial painting unfold before their eyes, while listening to the rhythmic sound of waves breaking over the reef. It is as if musical notes were carried by bubbling sounds rushing toward the shoreline.

In this humble propped house against the ocean, my fatherless family lived, consisting of seven siblings, my mother, and grandmother. Considered financially poor, we suffered many hardships. Yet, with the help of our grandmother, my siblings and I learned to be self-sufficient and became rich in heart by our environment. The sea provided us with a meager income, sufficient for school supplies and other necessities to survive. The coral reef supplied us with other nutritional foods, such as seaweed, clams, crustaceans, and other edible delectables. For our enjoyment, we made our own toys, playing games in the sand under the moonlight and reading books for our school assignments under the flickering light of a lamp. All of these experiences gave us the strength, supported by our faith, to grow and strive for a better future.

This is the place where I acquired my desire to learn, study, and understand the world of living things. My interests included core science subjects such as zoology, botany, chemistry, human anatomy, physiology, and microbiology. The fascination and inquisitiveness about conception and childbearing started at a very early age. My mother was a midwife by trade, bringing me along to her exhibitions around the villages. I carried her midwife kit provided by government healthcare programs and visited mothers-to-be and new mothers. I watched and learned as my mother gave them comfort, oil massages, and checked the newborn babies.

Being around my mother captivated and initiated my interest about the science of pregnancy. I retained all the information my mother indirectly taught me, including all the things that I read, watched, observed, and experienced over the years. These early experiences enabled me to consolidate my thoughts, and compile a book like this, especially during a time when information is readily available for reference whenever it is needed. That time is now.

Although, it has been difficult to formulate my thoughts over time, especially since I have been speaking about it for years, this needs to be written and further discussed. The process gave me the courage to express my innermost feelings through theoretical writing. I wanted to write it for a long time. So, the main goal of this book is to establish a module in a nonpartisan manner for the adversaries as well as sponsors for the abstinence method and/or the contraceptive method, while providing a meaningful, true, and proper practice. The controlled method and absticulate method are two methods designed to standardize a precise time table for teens and men to use as a guideline for effective orientation of—The Natural Uncharted Art of Lovemaking—in terms of conceiving, prevention of pregnancy, and childbirth spacing.

The methods can be instilled in every adolescent, single person, and married couple's mind repeatedly as a reminder for achieving their oriented goals. These concepts can be used to educate future generations as well. For example, it is no less important than other health and safety issues to become the priority of every company in order to insure effective production. It is a must for every company to reduce the never-ending increasing costs of health-related problems, underperformance productivity issues, and other costs associated with unsafe acts. As a company provides safe work and health environments using different health and safety modules to educate each and every employee, society should ensure effective solutions for pregnancy and prevention by educating teens and adults about sex and sexuality through these models.

This book will provide a natural concept to act as a buffer zone to educate adult singles, married couples, and teens about their own health and health safety, like sexually transmitted diseases (STDs) and/or pregnancy prevention. In regards to abstinence and contraceptives, women in particular are the ones who are pressured to use man-made contraceptive devices, some of which are known to contribute to women's health irregularities and/or complications over time. Contraceptives are often associated with the promotion of promiscuity, since taking birth control pills and such will hinder unwanted pregnancies.

For some men who practice abstinence, these concepts are a prelude that can contribute to misunderstandings, arguments, jealousy, or any other negative thoughts that can breed unhealthy habitual behaviors for every couple. It promotes sexual habits of self or mutual satisfaction, and increases a very high risk of conceiving during copulation without knowing the time that a woman's ovulation may occur. Men, in particular, while the body is at rest, keep producing sperm cells until ejaculation is performed. These sperm cells may even ooze out during a dream state. This is called a "wet dream." This type of dream still baffles many psychiatrists today. However, this phenomenon in man is not enough to deplete well stocked sperm cells.

Many highly educated people and many religious groups endorse abstention, but it is not a complete process. Because the male reproductive system is not like a female's reproductive system, the act of abstinence may in fact cause the opposite function. In this book, we will discuss the sexual behavior of adolescent males during adult maturation. It is impossible for a man to not discharge his sperm cells for a long period of time. It is not very realistic or natural for men to abstain from sex because the man's biological system is not mapped out or modeled to interfere with sperm production. The truth is, even married couples practice the taboos of sexual desires in their own particular ways. As men grow older and reach their upper 50s, this practice of men, which perceived by many as an unhealthy practice, will dissipate gradually until the golden age of man. Though many men may ignore condoms, they provide good protection against STDs, especially among promiscuous people and those trying to prevent impregnation. This book provides simple instructions which are easy to understand for everyone. By adhering to and following the guidelines proposed, individuals may become aware, perhaps merely enlightened, or amused by the different schemes on conception, pregnancy prevention, and childbirth spacing that can be viewed and performed.

Chapter One

CONTROLLED METHOD

Chapter One

CONTROLLED METHOD

❂

The controlled method is a technique to control the body's natural sexual desire. It is the ability of a man to subdue or stimulate his passion to engage in sexual intimacy in relation to conceiving, prevention of pregnancy, and childbirth spacing. It also acts to hinder the physiological, instinctive, sensational, and sexual behavior of man's complex wishful thinking.

This method is designed to outline segmented areas of the woman's menstrual cycle such as: the last 3 days of her menstrual cycle, her red zone area, ovulation area, buffer zone area, post-ovulation area, and free zone areas. These timeframes are useful to control a man's assertive sexual behavior. The idea is formed to orchestrate a compassionate atmosphere, an instrument to plot a precise and accurate practical calendar scheduling procedure.

The proposal is a revision popularized by Georgetown University in 1999. At that time, it was developed as a "new calendar-based fertility awareness method using a color-coded cycle beads method indicating infertile and fertile days of the menstrual cycle." The calendar-based, color-coded cycle beads were also a revision from a calendar-based method by a Roman Catholic physician from The Netherlands, who first formalized this method in 1930. But according to Stacy Wiegman, an editor for Bella Online Conception: "This method has limitations. It is just a calendar method by counting days...and avoiding intercourse on fertile days...although no research has been conducted to see how effective the standard days' method is in helping couples who are trying to conceive. It only helps pinpoint fertile days and infertile days and cycle length."

There is no exact way to pinpoint ovulation areas of the menstrual cycle, or when, and on what days ovulation may actually occur. Even if there is an exact science to pinpoint the fertile days and ovulation days of a woman, there is no way a woman can conceive or predict correctly when that may occur without the contribution of the man's sperm cells. A sperm cell is needed to fertilize one egg cell(s).

In any event, calendar scheduling is especially useful in industrialized countries and is very important in one's daily life. It affects everyone, including all living things in this world, where time is essential and the most crucial part of human existence. For example, "Plants uses circadian clocks to detect days. During the fall season, they produce seeds and drop their leaves. In spring, they grow flowers or fruits. During sunrise, they raise their leaves for photosynthesis for necessary nutrients, then in the evening, fold their leaves to prevent loss of moisture," according to the Genetic Learning Center, University of Utah. In people's lives, a set schedule is a designated time commitment to follow through, and it can be broken at any time when something very important comes up. Prioritizing our time schedule is necessary to maintain our daily undertakings. Sometimes in many industrialized countries, most adults think that time is too fast or it's too short.

On a day-to-day basis, time management is a recipe to reinforce our obligation between ourselves, with our loved ones, and in work. That is why man has to control himself in a timely manner to implement objectives and make decisions based solely on what is best.

This approach provides a tool to ensure that every opportunity is taken to implement effective timelines. In a general sense, time is one of the very important aspects of conceiving. When a woman reaches puberty, she will start to menstruate as a sign of maturity. It is a signal that her body's physiology is changing. She experiences enlargement of her breasts for milk storage, a sign that her body is ready for motherhood. This phenomenon is involuntary and accomplished without her control until the woman reaches her menopausal period (between 45 to 50 years of age), which is when the ovaries stop producing egg cells.

In today's modern world, we have developed a deep appreciation of technological advancements. We have mind-boggling information right at our fingertips, and nonstop voices on television programs, radio shows, advertisements, and commercials catching our attention, telling us how to make our body as well as mind healthy and how to live a "fulfilling" life. Sometimes, however, life's disappointments preoccupy our minds. Instinct becomes doubted and questioned, because it is overshadowed with negative visions of mirror images of "what if's". It seems that we no longer appreciate the mechanics of our thought processes. This negativity can shroud trust, reliance, and confidence, and adversely affect our personal expression, and eventually our interpersonal relationships.

The breath of dawn gives us a new beginning to strengthen our outlook on a new day. All the adverse, complex and unforeseeable stresses of life are always on our shoulders to carry, but a new day always has a different meaning that directly changes the quality of our daily life. The need to improve, to embrace new ideas and opportunities by transforming them into a positive viewpoint connect all efforts to capture the visual rhythm of conception. There is no secret that thoughtful understanding is necessary, and an exceptional dedication to each other will nourish intimate relationships.

When an intimate relationship is at the highest level, human instinct gravitates in setting aside time each day to share and listen to each other's ideas and eliminate questions and misunderstandings. This is important in order to minimize mistakes that are made and that our scheduled framework of goals and objectives are accomplished. It is very important to have a clear vision of what we wish to achieve in conjunction with a realistic expectation and assumption prior to beginning the technique and following the guidelines of the art of conceiving. This process is not an ordinary day-to-day procedure. When it is done properly, it can be accomplished with much pleasure and elevated to its true glory and rightful place among the cross-curriculum of arts and science.

This technique is an observable characteristic of man alone. Through understanding and careful observation of the male's reproductive system, we can see how man's physiological senses of the body will function in a very controlled environment in regards to having sexual intimacy with a woman. It is time to understand the importance of women and men's behavior and characteristics that contribute to the art of conception: the man's ability to prepare the body and mind and his physical energy to abstain or hold on or release his well-stocked sperm cells for conception, prevention of pregnancy, and childbirth spacing.

The woman's ovulation area or timeframe is traditionally the subject of many research studies without the contribution of man's respective observable characteristics. A man is always taken for granted that he can provide the necessary elements to impregnate egg cell(s) any time during female ovulation. This is just an underestimated, imaginary concept of females that is not actually true in many ways. Men are always flexible to perform these tasks. However, women and men need to be educated about the male reproductive system, conception contribution, pregnancy prevention influence, self and mutual-satisfaction, as well as woman's menstrual cycle.

Chapter Two

THE ART OF CONCEIVING

THE ART OF CONCEIVING

THE ART OF CONCEIVING

⊂═✦⊷

A t the present time, the subject of conception demands more attention than ever before. Many gifted men and women around the world have eagerly devoted their careers and time to figure out how they can help distressed, childless women conceive naturally. Natural conception, in my view, can be considered as one of the greatest of arts, but this art was pushed aside to the back burner in favor of technological advancements in scientific methods, especially in a time when women are favoring later-aged pregnancies due to professional opportunities. Everyone, especially men, can be arrogant, thinking that they are knowledgeable about conception and may contemplate seeking self-fulfillment much of the time in order to fulfill their sexual hunger.

First, man has to meticulously educate himself about his natural observable capabilities in order to perform at the highest level of lovemaking, and know by heart their female partner's menstrual cycle. This type of art is a science within itself. It is a reflection of what we are, which enables us to fulfill our way of life.

Second, perfecting the art requires a knowledge and understanding of your partner's character. It is an interactive love, self-confidence, patience, affection, tenderness, care, a warm embrace, devotion, and other positive senses that can permeate into mutually expansive traits of humanity that instinctually stimulate delightful pleasure for both parties. These traits are all integral parts or ingredients in developing passionate reflexes with even simple step-by-step instructions to improve and spark interest with great confidence to initiate lovemaking.

Men should understand that they are not only sperm donors, but true partners in the process. They should follow the appropriate principles to provide the highest degree of conception. When sperm cells are depleted to the very minimum, the body's physiological energy is also weakened to receive electrical impulses from the brain, which can impair sexual performance. It is very important to rest the body in order to replenish spent energy for sperm production. This type of activity is the most integral part of the male's responsibility.

As a general rule, men must be knowledgeable to recognize certain facts about a woman's menstrual cycle. In normal situations, a woman's monthly menstruation or "period" is usually on a 28-day cycle (plus or minus 2 days) before she starts the next cycle. How about the life span of an egg cell(s) after it settles itself within the lining of the fallopian tube walls? Is a man aware of this without definitive information? Egg cells are alive and well, like any other living thing in this world. There's time to be born, a time to grow in maturity, and a time to die.

When a woman menstruates, her cycle may not occur regularly. It may be shorter than 28 days, or longer, more or less than 5 days. This actual event is a necessity to purify her reproductive system in preparation for pregnancy. In this stage, egg cells are produced in the ovary, released downwards toward the fallopian tube. It moves in the darkness of the woman's body, and then mysteriously adheres to the thickened lining of the fallopian tube, forming a dimple-like indentation where some egg cell(s) settle themselves in a carefree environment. Other egg cell(s) are washed away during the menstrual cleansing process. Generally, this takes 3 days to complete this process. The egg cell(s) in the wall of the fallopian tube are then ready to be impregnated.

On the 4th day to the 14th day of the cycle, ovulation may actually occur in this particular area, but where? *Refer to "Chart I: Exhibit A, Guidelines of Conceiving III: Ovulation Area."*

In this area of the ovulation period, women begin to feel physiological urges and may become sexually active and motivated, making themselves attractive in order to catch the eye of the opposite sex. They bloom like flowers, spreading their scent to advertise their readiness to receive "pollen" in their natural habitat. Pollen carriers like bees collect nectar from flowers. They are prevalent in the wild. The wind also carries pollen to travel great distances to pollinate flowers to form seeds for their own generational cycle. This is just one example that can compare a blooming flower and ovulating woman. Bees, the wind, and pollen illustrate the nature of man.

In this segment of the menstrual cycle, somehow, a woman's most appealing characteristic is the way she walks with high heels on, swaying her hips side to side every step of the way, enticing man's attention. She is like a model walking on a runway platform during a modeling presentation. Her movements are composed of pretentious signals activating man's consciousness. She may feel like the prettiest woman in the world. Her confidence, hairstyle, and makeup are important and make her stand out to look and feel elegant. Naturally, during her fertile period, she makes herself attractive, is flirtatious, bold, outgoing, and confident to catch a man's attention. She takes pleasure in accentuating her attractiveness and is graceful in the man's eye. She is animated with a glowing aura to get noticed. Her lips are sensual. Her thin- or thick-arched eyebrows and curled eyelashes make her eyes mysterious. The magical magnetism of her eyes is intense and warm to induce and stimulate man's subconscious mind. Historically, even in biblical times, women magnify their natural beauty, using minerals, perfume, oil, and eyeliner to improve their appearance, like the big cats in the wild. Their hairstyle is arranged in such a way and is adorned with jewels and other ornaments to enhance their positive facial features. These characteristics during her fertile period are subconsciously performed.

In many instances, once a woman's ovulation is over, she tends to bring back her natural beauty. She is still graceful, free from awkwardness, communicates with feminine movements, is polite and attentive without letting her eyes wander, is confident and self-conscious, and her sexuality returns to a baseline modest mode.

Contrary to popular belief, it is time to begin or try something new with inspired imagination. Men often think that every successive release of his sperm contains a sufficient count of viable sperm to fertilize an egg cell(s). This belief about men is not true at all, not in science or in nature. Living things like the animals—sea mammals, birds, fish, insects, and seed-producing plants—have some similar aspect of the reproductive system of humans. All of them know how and when the right moment is to engage in intimacy to ensure future generational offspring.

However, it seems that more and more, women are becoming reliant on medicinal enrichment and other nutritional supplements to improve their chances to conceive. All of these anxieties are basically in the hands of women to control. Women are the only ones who can decide when to conceive or not to conceive by regulating men's ejaculation. To do this, there should be a set of rules or guidelines to minimize and optimize men's sperm production at any time, at any moment. Concurrently, both sexes are to mutually agree and understand the necessity to implement the planning of parenthood.

Chapter Three

CHART I: CONCEIVING

Chapter Three

CHART I: CONCEIVING

⊂═══⋊⊷

<u>**WOMAN'S**</u> MENSTRUAL CYCLE: NORMAL

Last 3 days of menstruation
Days

26. ⎤
27. ⎬ 3 days before menstruation
28. ⎦ Ovary produces egg cell(s)

Menstruation in progress
Day

1.

2.   RED ZONE AREA
            (Menstruation in progress)
3.

OVULATION AREA
Day

4.

5.

6.

7.

8.

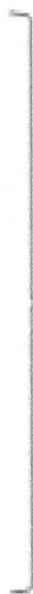

9.   CRITICAL AREAS

10.

11.

12.

13.

14.

BUFFER ZONE
Day
15.

POST-OVULATION AREA

16.
17.   POSITIVE/NEGATIVE AREAS
18.
19.

20.
21.
22.
23.   FREE ZONE
24.
25.

RULES OF CONCEIVING:

Women must:

- Aggressively regulate the enforcement of rules and guidelines.
- Have the ability to practice at the right moment.
- Set goals to implement confidence with each other.
- Be aware of the avoidable risk involved.
- Fulfill each other's duties using good judgment.
- Use common sense.
- Encourage and complement each other.
- Maintain healthy practices.
- Seek medical assistance when needed.

"EXHIBIT A" GUIDELINES OF CONCEIVING: Normal

I. LAST 3 DAYS OF MENSTRUATION CYCLE

DAYS: 26, 27, & 28

MAN:

- Man must know and gauge (with help of the woman) the first day of menstruation to ensure the exact calendar scheduling.
- Man must start to abstain from sexual activity at least 3 days before the menstrual cycle starts to ensure quality sperm production.

WOMAN:

- ✓ Egg cell(s) are old, physiological impulse starts to trigger egg cell production.
- ✓ The ovary releases egg cell(s) moving at a very minute pace toward the fallopian tubes.
- ✓ The fallopian tube linings and the old, unfertilized egg cell(s) start to shed off, cleansing and purifying the body in preparation for pregnancy.

II. RED ZONE AREA

DAY 1, 2, & 3-4

MAN:

Men must continue to abstain and maintain quality sperm production so that they can build up a mature, strong, healthy sperm count until the time to release the sperm with a high degree of impregnating an egg cell. This 7-day window of abstaining from sexual activity without ejaculation will ensure a quality and sufficient supply of sperm cells with the proper pressure buildup and proper erectile of the penis to execute a precise trajectory of ejected sperm to reach the egg cell(s) in the fallopian tubes.

WOMAN:

On Day 1, the menstrual cycle and flow begins. The fallopian tubes start to swell, forming dimple-like diminutive indentations along the lining of the wall where egg cell(s) adhere and settle down. Some egg cells are washed away along with menstrual fluids. Some egg cell(s) settle down in their purified environment. This process takes 2 to 3 days to take place. The first 2 to 3 days are bloody, so practice cleanliness. Conceiving in this area is positively possible. Egg cell(s) are ready for impregnation.

III. OVULATION AREA: Normal

DAY 4-5, 6, 7, 8, 9, 10, 11, 12, 13, & 14

MAN:

With proper preparation of the body and mind, this area is the most critical segment of the menstrual cycle, where ovulation may actually occur. In order to cover all the areas where ovulation may actually happen (without the aid of some costly devices like pregnancy kits or other devices), man must initiate vaginal sexual intercourse every 48 hours or more or every other day, but not less than 48 hours to maintain an adequate supply of mature, healthy, strong sperm cells to replace the weakened sperm and thus, penetrate the egg cell(s). Excessive ejaculation depletes a man's sperm count. Again, sexual intercourse must be done every 2 days but not less than 48 hours to ensure maintaining an adequate supply of strong sperm to swim up to, reach, and be able to fertilize one egg cell.

WOMAN:

OVULATION DAYS: Normal

DAYS—(1st month):	DAYS—(2nd month):
5. *	4. *
6.	5.
7. *	6. * Note: Adjust 1 or 2 days if the clearing of
8.	7. the menstrual bloody fluid is over 4 days.
9. *	8. * Then wait for clearing. Adjust your calendar
10.	9. intercourse schedule.
11. *	10. *
12.	11.
13. *	12. *
14.	13.
	14. *

(*) Indicate trial days. (Scheduled vaginal intercourse day)

IV. BUFFER ZONE

Day 15

MAN & WOMAN:

This day is to be considered as the neutral zone, the positive and negative area of the ovulation. Female egg cell(s) are rubbery and bouncy, making it difficult for the male sperm to penetrate its cell wall. The egg cell(s) are old and matured. The chance of conceiving is still possible, depending if the menstrual fluid is beyond normal clearing.

V. POST- OVULATION AREA

DAYS 16, 17, 18, & 19 – Positive/Negative Areas

WOMAN:

Positive/negative areas. Chance of conceiving is still possible, depending if the menstrual fluid is beyond normal clearing. The chance of conceiving in this area drops day-by-day to a very minimum level to none.

DAYS 20, 21, 22, 23, 24, & 25 – Free Zone

WOMAN:

Free zone areas. The woman's body's physiological impulses start to transmit impulses to the ovaries for egg cell(s) production, triggers the menstrual cycle. The ovary will burst to release new egg cell(s) to start the menstrual cycle.

VI. MENSTRUAL CYCLE BEGINS: 2nd month

On the first day of menstruation, always start counting for the proper calendar scheduling. In a normal situation, menstrual fluids start to clear up after the third or fourth day, so initiate the first trial at the 4th or 5th day whenever possible. A man must have at least a minimum of 48 hours of an old stock of sperm cells. Whenever possible, do not deviate from the norm. Follow the guidelines precisely and practice good judgment and good hygiene.

Personal Experience:

In 1978, this idea was born out of extraordinary beginning. It was broadened with deep analysis many years later with the male's ability to control sperm production and ejaculation. These two characteristics of men go hand in hand with a woman's capability to conceive.

From personal experiences around mid-March 1978, I took my wife and my newborn twin sons home from the hospital when we were surprised to find some visitors waiting on the doorsteps of our apartment. It was my childhood relative, Marina, who I've never seen since high school and her husband, Harry. We were happy, talking about our childhood days, growing up in a rural, poor fishing village of the northern Philippines. It was a joy meeting her husband and introduce them to my wife.

During our conversation, Harry asked me what method we used to end up having twins. I thought he was joking, but he then revealed that he and Marina were married for over 5 years and have been unsuccessful in conceiving a child. He told me that a doctor confirmed that he was impotent, and thus, unable to impregnate his wife. Not satisfied with the results of his test, he sought a second opinion to confirm the previous clinical results. A few months later, to his surprise and dismay, the second doctor also confirmed that he was indeed unable to produce enough viable sperm. He desperately wanted to create a family, and do his part as a man to help his wife conceive. At that time as a new dad and husband, what was I to say to a fellow husband and longing potential father? I was dumbfounded.

I asked him if he had sexual intimacy with his wife the night before he went to the doctors for the test. He admitted that he did, in fact, have sexual intercourse twice the night before his appointments, hoping his wife would get pregnant. I thought the test results were odd, so I told him with hopeful confidence, "I think you still have a chance to get your wife pregnant." Hearing this, his eyes flew open with a gleam of optimism, and he smiled.

After our lunch together, I traced back a memory about what a previous university professor said, "Beware if the sperm is a yellowish cream color." This was the beginning of my thoughts about how to help women who are having difficulties conceiving. It is necessary to understand how to prepare, both, a man's and a woman's body in order to be able to conceive. I did a bit of reviewing from my past both educational and life experience, and followed up with Harry and Marina. I spoke with them about a detailed plan on how and when to have sexual intimacy. I warned him not to deviate from this method and remain dedicated at least for a few months. Three months later, Marina was pregnant with their first child. Less than two years later, their second child was born. Today, they are blessed with two wonderful daughters to carry their legacy.

A few months after Harry and Marina's news, my wife and I decided that she would stop using contraceptive pills and be more open to using this technique. This I explained that it centered on her rhythmic menstrual calendar and schedule. Our goal was to create a space between my twin sons and another child using natural prevention methods without contraceptives. Five years later, as planned, we were blessed with a daughter. At first, it was risky, but we diligently practiced natural prevention to reduce any chance for my wife to get become pregnant again. It took a lot of courage and determination to practice natural preventative methods without using contraceptives.

I have been sharing this method for at least 34 years now with many married couples who were having difficulties conceiving. I shared my advised plan and opinions regarding this style of conception and how to prevent pregnancies. These people have been my family, extended relatives, friends, friends of friends, and coworkers. Now I would like to share this concept beyond my inner cycle of family and friends.

Another friend expressed his concern about his brother who had just recently got married. He thought he might not be able to father a child because as a boy, one of his testicles did not fully develop and drop. So I told my friend that I wanted to talk to his brother about my conception method. Eventually, I had a chance to talk to his brother and told him to have faith in God and himself, and with God's blessing, he would father a child as long as he followed the process that I would share with him. I told him to try my method for at least 3 months before he sought medical help. On his first try, his wife became pregnant with a daughter. I eventually became the godfather to his only child.

Sometimes unfortunate events are the only time people are brought together; from death, comes life. At a friend's funeral, I met with my niece and her husband, who I have not seen since their wedding over a year ago. I teasingly asked them, "No bambino yet?" Both became embarrassed and speechless. Tactfully, I opened up about sharing with them about my ideas about how to conceive. This was the time when my niece's husband privately opened up that he might have difficulties or even be unable to father a child because he was treated for cancer when he was younger. I told him to have faith, but he cut me off by saying, "I don't believe in the religious aspect of life." I simply told him, "Have faith in YOURSELF. Create a positive approach, and do not deviate from this method and schedule." Eight months later, I saw them at my brother's birthday party. I saw her turn the corner with her rounded tummy. I found out that her delivery date was in a couple of weeks. We exchanged laughs and congratulations.

In 2011, a coworker of mine indicated to me that she and her husband have been trying to have a second child for 5 years. Both sought professional help by going to a doctor for consultations, but had no luck at all. So she ended up buying the recommended expensive fertility kit to monitor her ovulation period, but nothing worked. So one day, I built up the courage to talk to her about my method and told her that if she will follow it, she may be successful conceiving. I told her that she will be the one to control their scheduled lovemaking and her husband's ejaculation and be committed to the process. On their first attempt a month later, she immediately conceived. Nine months later, a baby boy was born, followed with another pregnancy a couple of months later.

Another time during my lunch break at work, some of my coworkers started to joke around about different issues such as politics, work-related issues, family issues, and eventually, pregnancy. One of the men mentioned that after a few years of married life, he has no child yet. One day, I saw him during his lunch break by himself, so I joined him for my short coffee break. He was receptive to me communicating with him about this idea. So, I devised a plan for him to follow and assured him that everything would be all right if he tried the method as I outlined it. This conversation took place late 2011. I told him to try this method in beginning of the year during his wife's ovulation period. Whenever I saw him after that, I never mentioned it anymore.

Around mid-March, I asked him, "How's it going? Has the method worked?" To my delight, he informed me that his wife was already in her first trimester of pregnancy. He was reluctant to tell me about it because his wife almost had a miscarriage. He was so joyful, and happy about being a father-to-be. In the fall of 2012, during our coffee break he excitedly and proudly showed everyone the picture of his baby daughter born just a few days ago. He had his biggest smile. We all extended our hands in congratulatory handshakes.

These events are the main reason why I have chosen to write this manuscript. Regardless of what people have speculated or jokingly remarked, the proposed method may inform others to think differently about conception and intercourse, directly or indirectly. If this topic begins the conversation and dialogue among couples and/or friends, I have contributed somehow. Like a baby's birth, it is a seed borne out of extraordinary beginnings

Most people only understand the basic concept of pregnancy. They only understand that when a woman menstruates, it produces egg cells, and a man expels and produces sperm cells, that, when combined through sexual intercourse, produces a pregnancy. This is quite true, but much more is involved in how to conceive and how to prevent pregnancies without using contraceptives which can help us to achieve our goals that are influenced or affected by economics and status.

Chapter Four

THE ART OF PREVENTION

Chapter Four

THE ART OF PREVENTION

⊂═⋆⊳

Prevention is an act to avoid human unintentional errors caused by unconscious or cognizant carelessness. Regardless of what we do in life, even a slight deviation from safe practices can be detrimental to our health and safety, as well as that of others. Human mistakes are made by poor judgment and a lack of concentration. This is also true within the context of family planning.

A cornerstone in love-making is to engage in safe, natural practices, good hygiene, and rational behavior that ensures and supports safe, sexual, natural habits. These behaviors are critical for making ethical decisions without guilt. When possible, try to follow the right approach and make the best decision; however, even a slight error in doing so may result in repercussions that cannot be corrected.

This concept addresses the most basic form of natural pregnancy prevention. It is the result of an in-depth analysis of man's behavior and characteristics. It promotes education, understanding, and cooperation in order to accomplish the objectives of this method designed for birth control.

First of all, a man must have a thorough understanding in regards to a woman's concern about whether or not to conceive. Awareness and ethical decisions are the main foundation to prevent unwanted pregnancies from occurring. Insufficient knowledge and carelessness can cause unintentional mistakes to happen, and risk recognition is critical for accuracy in performing the responsible act of prevention. Poor judgment can damage self-confidence.

Second, pregnancy prevention is really challenging to accomplish naturally, especially with adolescents. By knowing all the risks involved, it becomes the man's responsibility to overcome and control his assertive behavior. He always has the desire to initiate sexual intimacy and not pay close attention to his duty to avoid conception. It is the woman's responsibility to determine if she is ready and open to conceive or not, and it is the man's duty to comply with her decision. Open communication is necessary between partners for conceiving, prevention and child-birth spacing.. Miscommunication in combination with irresponsible intercourse may lead to awkwardness, a downward spiral of misjudgment, misunderstanding of true feelings and intentions, and as far as unwanted propagation and/or abortion. A man's personal interests might impair the relationship's objective, and he might make decisions based solely for his own benefit. Therefore, every woman must aggressively enforce her rules and guidelines to minimize human error which results from not following proper procedures.

Society is geared to influence opinion and challenge thoughts, and indirectly forces change in our courses of action. People fail to remember that change begins within us, our freedom to choose. To change one's perspective is to develop and explore other possibilities that can improve our ways of thinking instead of merely basing our thinking on tradition, which can be at odds with the lightning-fast changing world we live in. Unfortunately, we focus on protectionism, insecurities, and restrictions, which impede cooperation for implementation and practice for sexually-motivated natural methods. Our experiences and religious beliefs dictate our behaviors, including the taboos that we subscribe to and that influence us.

(A). THE "ABSTICULATE METHOD"

This method is a universal practice that can no longer be denied or ignored by educated people. Most of the time, people hesitate to speak freely about certain matters, especially the taboos of sexual desires and certain personal practices. People are generally private about this. Most mature people tend to suppress this, deny it, or fail to express their ideas about it. For example, the word "masturbate" has a very unpleasant and unhealthy connotation to everyone. It can symbolize immoral values and behaviors. However, this behavior is acceptable to practice in clinics around the world to provide sperm count samples, for sperm banking, and for in vitro fertilization. Cinema has also glorified this act among women for personal pleasure. Nonetheless, masturbation is a taboo to educate men and women about the proper usage of this practice for the prevention of pregnancy and childbirth spacing.

Many educated people encourage the use of modern man-made contraceptives, and others have a special interest in more government funding at the expense of taxpayers to spread the use of these devices for economic reasons. Instead of using government-allocated funding for child development education, good nutrition, and appropriate school educational materials, we have allowed sex videos to be shown to many students in classrooms across the United States.

If this word "masturbate" can be eloquently verbalized into a deeper definition to include abstinence, it can be expressed as "ABSTICULATE." This word has a richer meaning to express its thought.

ABSTICULATE—IS A WORD DERIVED FROM TWO ROOT WORDS: ABSTAIN and EJACULATE

It is a natural method to abstain from vaginal sexual intercourse without depriving the body of sexual desire by way of sperm ejaculation through mutual or self-masturbation, and oral or anal sex.

This method emphasizes the naturalness of human desire and promotes abstinence. However, it is associated with substandard knowledge about the true meaning of abstinence. Because of the lack of knowledge, man himself becomes the biggest contributor to all teen pregnancies and other unwanted pregnancies because of his desire to "score" with the woman and his unwillingness to avoid taking risks.

It is necessary and essential to educate everyone from puberty to adulthood that natural practices are normal indeed, especially when contraceptive devices are not readily available. Educational guidelines should include the "ABSTICULATE METHOD" to promote and/ or compliment the real meaning of abstinence, instead of avoiding this subject, making it a taboo to every parent, educators, healthcare professional researchers, politicians, and others. They state that this method is not appropriate to formally educate junior high school, high school, and even university-level students. Thus, allowing the passing on misguided or ill-informed use of masturbation from parent to child or student to student. How can these groups of people deprive young, mature men and women about the facts of life and the body's sexual desires that include: lust, desire, longings, cravings, hunger, thirst, passion, wishes, appeals, and hopes, since young people use this system from puberty through adulthood and married life? Isn't it hidden away within the comfort of one's bedroom readily available to experience anytime? Or, do we just let teens in particular learn about it and practice it themselves without proper guidance, because it will come out naturally? Why hasn't this type of abstinence ever been academically introduced to educate young men and women, mature singles, and married couples, especially families with more than one child, about the true meaning of "abstain" in its natural form?

Instead, these people only look for the easy way out, always asking the government to set aside funds for the promotion and implementation of man-made manufactured contraceptive devices, which may affect a women's health over time. Condoms, in particular, are acceptable for the prevention of sexually transmitted diseases for many promiscuous people, but as the label reads, 'not 100% preventable against conception'.

This method is a system that should be introduced as the first defense for birth control. Men and women must both embrace the concept of the "Absticulate Method" twice within 48 hours before vaginal intercourse as a moral obligation to ensure the depletion of strong viable sperm cells before vaginal intercourse. This method is 99.9 percent pure as gold. It involves the removal of impurities in the body's sexual desire through the understanding of man's physiological impulses. It provides focus, good judgment, and common sense. Both men and women can set goals to reinforce the ability to practice this method in a timely manner, and become more aware of the risks involved. To prove that this method is accurate, first, man should know about his body's ability to produce sperm cells after two successive ejaculations within a 2-day period, and what is the nature of semen on the third ejaculation, as long as it is not longer than 48 hours.

Second, man must check with a doctor to see to if his sperm count is at the normal threshold level after two successive ejaculations. The only drawback is, at the clinic, the egos of men may suffer when asked to masturbate behind curtains or in a bathroom stall in order to provide a sperm sample for a sperm count analysis. If the count is below the normal threshold, the man will be declared impotent.

Man has always been a macho show-off, flexing his muscles indicating his superiority to "perform" and eventually impregnate a woman at anytime, anywhere, and whenever he may feel like it. No matter who he is, whether the Incredible Hulk, Superman, Mr. Universe, a Democrat or Republican, the town mayor or councilman, a principal or teacher, doctor or lawyer, rich or poor, even Jack standing with his female friend, Rose, at the railing of the *Titanic* spitting out a ball of his saliva as he challenges his friend to see whose spit will reach the farthest, he will deplete his stock of saliva upon successive occasions. This is just one example to correlate man's ability to ejaculate for the third consecutive time within the allowable time limit.

Once a man executes the "Absticulate Method" twice within 48 hours, he no longer has enough sperm in the semen to ejaculate the third time, and it will be hard and take longer to achieve a climax. His sperm will be too immature and too weak to swim up to reach and fertilize an egg cell(s). That is why honesty, mutual understanding, monitoring the time, and scheduling of a man's ejaculation are the tools a woman can make use of before engaging in sexual intercourse.

This "Absticulate Method" is the best form of a natural method. It is the most effective one and costs nothing to prevent pregnancy. It is very important to implement this method in unconditional lovemaking. This method has been practiced throughout the world. Unfortunately, no one wants to discuss this method; it is considered taboo outside of the bedroom. It is not a topic of open forum or public gatherings. It is avoided by parents and teachers, medical health professionals, religious leaders, government social researchers, lobbyists, politicians, and others. No one wants to raise this subject.

Many people believe that this type of prevention is a sexually motivated behavior that promotes sexual conduct. It is not brought up for open discussion because this method is considered improper. It is deemed discourteous to educate young adolescents about it. But when this method is used properly and young adolescents are educated about it, they can positively affect their future. They need to be properly educated about their biological sexual desires and sexual characteristics instead of learning it all by themselves through their experiences, without proper guidance from parents, educators, religious, and medical healthcare practitioners. Otherwise, it will cost the government in health and welfare services because of the high increase of teen and other unwanted pregnancies as well as consequences due these engagements. The investment for better education and practices in maternal and child health compete for societal attention and importance, which is hindered by increasing contraceptive distribution and subsidiary costs for unwanted pregnancies, like abortion. Even with rising allocated support from taxpayers to promote contraceptive devices rather than education first, these pregnancies and the social problems that accompany them will remain a prevalent problem in years to come.

Eventually, this practice will be introduced into the world as a primary or complimentary guideline for natural pregnancy prevention. This method can be conducted in such a way so as to neutralize negative concerns of many women regarding the use of modern contraceptives. The demand for women to use contraceptives may be prejudicial and biased. Women in particular may be used for the purpose of gathering statistical data to prove the validity of product, while men are more or less ignored and undereducated about their sexual desire toward women. In a general sense, most men are allowed to seek women for sexual satisfaction without any repercussions.

Contraceptives are designed to prevent pregnancy. However as expressed by most adults, it promotes promiscuity in teens and other women, while contributing to a higher probability of acquiring sexually transmitted diseases unless condoms are consistently used for men. In a monogamous relationship, there is no need to use modern contraceptives, but can be treated as an alternative or complimentary while practicing the "Absticulate Method."

On one hand, abstinence deprives the body's sexual emotional desire, which results in mutual or self-motivated satisfaction, such as oral or anal copulation. In other words, the individual(s) "absticulate." This practice is also used in the gay and lesbian communities around the world. This lifestyle has been a part of human existence ever since biblical times. Since this lifestyle is still taboo in the eyes of many, the individuals that practice it may establish a community to live and congregate freely as a group of people. Others are overwhelmed by prejudices and injustices so they choose to live secret lives. Typically, these communities provide comfort and acceptance for their members, where people feel relaxed and connected. Many of these individuals are motivated to live close together for their own safety in order to practice their own chosen sexual orientation without discrimination from others who are less tolerant.

Since abstinence is a natural part of the "Absticulate Method," it is time to take this issue out from bedrooms all around the country and use it as a tool to educate men and women, especially teens, as a birth control preventative. It is imperative to restructure family planning programs by the government to include the natural practices of abstinence. We need easy-to-understand instructional materials, pamphlets, and visual aids that include the "Absticulate Method" as a natural means of abstinence, in lieu of man-made contraceptive devices, which are very costly to the government. This method can be taught to students in junior high school up to the university level in a curriculum regarding human sexuality.

This idea should supersede or be included into some other educational materials that are being used today, like several semi-X-rated "educational" videos. The time that students spend watching these videos should be reduced unless deemed truly all-encompassing about sex and sexuality. Within the framework of the "Absticulate Method," a well-written book would be more informative than any of those videos that are currently being shown to students in classroom settings. A book of this nature, to prevent unwanted pregnancies, would be accepted across generational lines. Promotionally, modern contraceptive devices should be treated as an alternative for pregnancy prevention, and it should be encouraged as such.

(B). ABSTAIN METHOD

Abstinence is characterized by stopping sexual intercourse during the fertile days after a woman's menstrual cycle. This type of method is perceived by men as an intrusion in their sexual desire. It is too vague to comprehend, and it's too great to follow through. It also requires intermittent suppression of one's sexual desire which can turn into very limited sexual intercourse habits and might cause havoc in a relationship and provoke arguments. Repetitive abstinence can also interfere with the instinctive motor that drives the sexual senses of men. This notion is challenging to men, believe it or not.

To practice this method requires a strong commitment to carry out such a task. It involves man's will to execute his undeniable sexual desire to uphold family goals, traditions, and moral values. But this commitment, many times, can be broken when man's unquenchable hunger overpowers him, and he begins to succumb to his self-gratifying, irresistible sexual temptations.

Abstaining is one of the best methods for birth control, because of its 100% guarantee of no penetration, no sperm release, therefore no sperm-egg contact. But it is not the most realistic and the most desirable method to use for teens discovering their sexuality and others, whose mental will is not as strong as most. This method is still not enough to cover the whole scenario of abstinence.

This concept to prevent pregnancy has been endorsed for as long as the core rallying cry for many religious sects around the world. It seems to be a very good idea, but in real life, especially among male teens with raging hormones as well as men, it is unrealistic to believe that they can practice the abstaining method throughout their entire life without the support of an understanding friend or partner. For teens and women, it is still their choice to practice this method whenever needed, and quite a few of female teens practice this method and remain a virgin until they marry. The only questionable drawback is can these teens really practice abstinence to prevent pregnancy during their married life without contraceptive use? And how about the other groups of teens and women that contribute to the problems of teen and other unwanted pregnancies? So, men and women must be educated about the menstrual ovulation area of a woman and the sexual characteristics of man to practice the natural method.

CHART II: PREGNANCY PREVENTION AND CHILDBIRTH SPACING

WOMAN'S MENSTRUAL
CYCLE: NORMAL

MEN's ABSTICULATE
METHOD

**Last 3 days of
menstruation cycle**
Days
26. ⎤
27. ⎬ 3 days before
28. ⎦ menstruation Ovary
produces egg cell(s)

⎫
⎬ FREE ZONE
⎭

Menstruation in progress
Day
1. ⎤
2. ⎬ RED ZONE AREA
3. ⎦ (Menstruation in
progress)

OVULATION AREA
Day
4.
5.
6.
7.
8.
9. ⎬ CRITICAL AREAS
10. New egg cell(s)
11.
12.
13.
14.

⎫
⎬ Practice "Absticulate
⎭ Method" & good
judgment

WOMAN'S MENSTRUAL CYCLE: NORMAL	**MEN's** ABSTICULATE METHOD

BUFFER ZONE
Day
15.

POST-OVULATION AREA
16. ⌉
17. ⎬ POSITIVE/
18. ⎬ NEGATIVE AREAS
19. ⌋

20. ⌉
21. ⎪
22. ⎬ FREE ZONE
23. ⎪
24. ⎪
25. ⌋

FREE ZONE, Old
egg cells(s)

RULES OF PREVENTION:

MAN:

The key to prevention is for man to understand about a woman's menstrual cycle, regardless of an existence of a present partner. Understand the risk factors associated with conception. Practice self-control and encourage others to do what is right. Behave responsibly.

WOMAN:

A woman must enforce the rules of pregnancy prevention and follow the guidelines. She must be aware of her own cycle and be willing to communicate this with her partner.

FAMILIARIZATION OF MENSTRUAL CYCLE:

The last 3 days of the menstrual cycle, the ovary produces egg cell(s). The first 3 days, a natural involuntary phenomenon occurs without the woman's control. This involves the cleansing of the fallopian tubes to be purified in preparation for pregnancy. Egg cell(s) are released from the ovaries slowly into the fallopian tubes while the cleansing process is in progress. Egg cell(s) settle in the fallopian tube lining in a diminutive dimple-like indentation. The egg cell(s) are now ready for impregnation. A normal menstrual cycle will last 28 days. The first day of menstruation is very critical for the calendar-prevention scheduling.

EXHIBIT B: PREVENTION GUIDELINES:

I. RED ZONE AREA
DAY 1, 2, & 3-4

✓ Practice cleanliness. Conception is possible.

✓ Also, avoid sexual intercourse as much as possible in this area, and mutually agree with your partner to release mature, healthy, strong sperm cells by the "Absticulate Method" and perform responsibly.

II. OVULATION AREA
DAY 4-5, 6, 7, 8, 9, 10, 11, 12, 13, &14: Fertile Period

MAN:

This is the most critical area—practice self-control, be honest, trust, act responsibly, and make right decisions. Avoid sexual intercourse as much as possible. However, in case you do have intercourse, make sure to use the "Absticulate Method" twice within 48 hours to ensure depletion of the strong, healthy sperm cells before submitting to vaginal intercourse, in order to significantly decrease the chances of conception. Remember that with the man's third ejaculation, his body's physiological energy is too weak to receive electrical impulses from the brain to generate an intense drive to make love. At this moment, his penis is not fully erect. Without the proper pressure and proper erectile, it can only eject a small amount of anemic semen with weak and immature sperm cells. The trajectory power of the penis is not strong enough to reach the egg cell(s). Vaginal intercourse should be done at this time. Do not hold more than 48 hours of sperm cell stock. Use the "Absticulate Method" if necessary. Consistent and proper practices develop safer practices to prevent pregnancy. Be sure to perform responsibly and practice cleanliness.

WOMAN:

It is the woman's responsibility to continue to enforce the rules of pregnancy prevention and follow the guidelines.

III. BUFFER ZONE: The Positive and Negative Area of Ovulation:

Day 15

This day must be considered as a positive and negative area of ovulation. Practice precautionary measures in this area to prevent pregnancy because the chance of conceiving is still possible. Use the "Absticulate Method," if necessary. Avoid over 48 hours of sperm cell stock.

IV. SECOND PART: POST- OVULATION AREA
DAY 16, 17, 18, & 19

This is a FREE ZONE area. The chance of conceiving is still possible. Practice precautionary measures. The possibility of conception drops day by day to its lowest point during this time.

V. FREE ZONE
DAY 20, 21, 22, 23, 24, 25, 26, 27, & 28-29

VI. NEXT MENSTRUAL CYCLE—2ND MONTH

(C). MAN-MADE CONTRACEPTIVES:

CONDOM:

Around the world, condom usage is being widely encouraged to prevent sexually transmitted diseases (primarily), as well as pregnancies. The original concept of this device was supposed to function as a barrier to inhibit sperm cells to fertilize the egg cell(s), thus preventing pregnancy. However, with dreaded diseases like HIV (human immunodeficiency virus) or AIDS (acquired immune deficiency syndrome) so widespread, it became the primary mechanism to contain the spread of these diseases, as well as other diseases that can be acquired through sexual intercourse. Today, the condom is still used to prevent pregnancy as well as the spread of Sexually Transmitted Diseases.

It is important to keep in mind that whoever uses this device needs to practice sensible safe acts, and proper use of this device and the safe disposal of it is important to everyone and the environment. As usual, some promiscuous people will carelessly use this device infrequently for their own protection, but others who really need help, like families with multiple children and teens who want to prevent unwanted pregnancies, may find that it is not freely available to them, especially in poor and low socioeconomic communities where teen pregnancies and other unwanted pregnancies remain a problematic issue for the local government's healthcare system and social services. Although condoms are effective, they are still not widely used as the primary alternative for birth control, and are still being ignored by many, who wish for better alternatives like a natural method.

CONTRACEPTIVE PILLS and INTRAUTERINE DEVICE (IUD)

CONTRACEPTIVE PILLS and INTRAUTERINE DEVICE (IUD)

M ost married women in developed countries use contraceptive pills or IUDs for their family planning method for the purpose of preventing pregnancies. Highly educated single and married women continuously use these devices to avoid pregnancy in order to maintain their lifestyle and/or status quo. Undereducated single women or married women occasionally or inconsistently use these devices. However, medical science has evidence that these devices are having negative health side effects. Extended usage over months or even years may result in health problems. Many symptoms may not appear immediately.

The main drawback of these methods is cost over time. For those who have limited income, these methods can absorb a significant amount of the monthly budget. Unwanted pregnancies and women with multiple children are very common, especially in poor communities across the United States and the rest of the world, whether the countries are industrialized or developing. The only distinction is, in developed countries, there are governmental subsidies like health and welfare services to help ease and support those in need of these services. In other countries, there is no or limited budgetary funding, however meager, set aside to subsidize their growing national problems. Health care, welfare, education, and jobs cost money for every country, which can keep them from moving forward.

(D). OTHER FORMS of PREGNANCY PREVENTION:

TUBAL LIGATION and VASECTOMIES:

These methods are the ultimate form of pregnancy prevention. They are surgical procedures that can inhibit pregnancy. In industrialized countries where medical insurance is common to cover the cost of these surgical techniques, it is easy for married couples and often single parents with more than one child to obtain. They may not even have to spend a dime to undergo these surgeries. But mentally and psychologically, it may be very expensive for some couples and may be the hardest decision of their married life. Generally, however, any lingering negative thoughts will subside and fade away over time.

These surgical procedures require couples to deeply consider what they want in their family life. Mutual understanding and agreement is necessary to ease and overcome any undesirable negative thoughts so that they can have these procedures done without guilt or regret. Some forms are reversible, but consulting the physician about options is vital to the conversation.

(E). MODERN FORM OF CONCEIVING:

IN VITRO FERTILIZATION:

In vitro fertilization was conceptualized by the remarkable idea to develop a scientific way of fertilizing egg cells outside a woman's womb. This type of conception is performed with laboratory apparatus to achieve fertilization. It is an intricate process performed by physicians and technicians, especially those who specialize in fertility problems. This method of conception is a technological leap for mankind. This procedure is costly both, in money and time, and the success rate is still not at a level most couples hope for. Therefore, this procedure should be the last alternative to be administered for those who are eager to conceive a child.

According to the Advanced Fertility Center of Chicago, "The United States national average of in vitro fertilization live birth rates statistics for 2010 is 45% for less than 35 years old...as a woman ages, the success rate by using her own eggs starts to drop in the 20s, and drops faster in the mid-30s and early 40s...live births are rare at age 44 and above...there's no drop in the success rate with age when using young donor eggs."

(F). WOMEN'S IRREGULAR MENSTRUATION:

Many things can contribute to this phenomenon of a woman's menstrual cycle. There's nothing a couple can do but wait for the right moment when the next cycle of menstruation appears if she is irregular. For example, if the menstrual cycle appears for the month, and the menstrual fluid does not stop at the normal stage of 3 to 4 days, and went beyond, about 6 or 7 days, the possibility of conceiving is lower than normal because the egg cell(s) start to travel at the first day of the menstrual cycle, and it takes 3 days for the egg to travel from the ovary to the fallopian tube to adhere to its lining. It is possible that the egg cells could have washed away along with the menstrual fluids.

Assume that there are egg cell(s) which are strong enough to cling to the lining of the fallopian tube waiting to be impregnated; it is the man's responsibility to wait for menstrual clearing before lovemaking. Irregular menstruation involves missing a month or two of one's menstrual cycle, a normal problem of many women today. If this happens, wait for the next cycle of menstruation to appear, and wait for a normal clearing of menstrual fluids to dissipate before initiating lovemaking. Refer to the guidelines of conceiving *Exhibit A: III. OVULATION.* Remember that menstruation is a woman's physiological process to cleanse and purify the womb in preparation for conception. At least six menstrual cycle trials must be performed in an attempt to conceive before seeking professional medical help.

GLOBAL PERSPECTIVES:

Globally, on every continent and in all countries, there will be an increase or decrease in the population. One example of a nation experiencing an increasing population is the Philippines. It is a known fact that this nation's population is steadily climbing toward the 100 million mark. The government is struggling on how to slow down this alarming trend of a fast-rising population. Unless there is proper population control, this tendency will drag the economy down. The need of a natural preventative method is vitally necessary to educate the population on how to slow down this trend. Religion and a lack of sexual education have contributed to this disturbing trend.

In fact, to slow down this trend, a realistic natural family planning method to educate women and men from puberty onwards is urgently needed, rather than pushing the use of man-made manufactured contraceptive products as first line defense for prevention, such as condoms, birth control pills, IUDs, etc. These products should be used as a second alternative method to prevent pregnancy because of their expense and the difficulty of distribution to the whole population over time. It will also cost the government a substantial amount of money to implement distribution even for just a few years. To add to these problems, some of the devices require a medical prescription and the consent of doctors for them. If economics are a non-issue for couples or individuals, these methods may provide another technique to pair with current choices of prevention.

An IUD (Intrauterine Device) is a device that can prevent sperm from fertilizing an egg cell. This is a procedure that requires doctors to place the IUD properly in the woman's uterus during the ovulation period, and the possibility of negative side effects can occur.

Contraceptive pills can be costly over time, require a medical prescription, and only effective after a couple of months of use (not immediate). When used properly daily, they can effectively prevent pregnancy, but over time, they, too, have negative side effects.

Condoms are probably the best alternative device to promote pregnancy prevention because they also cover prevention of sexually transmitted diseases that can be acquired through sexual intercourse. Contrary to many congressmen/women who are proponents of the Reproductive Health Bill (a bill being introduced in the Philippines Congress for debate), if passed, reproductive health services throughout the country will be hard to implement because of funding problems associated with the distribution of such devices. Jobs, administration, educational materials, and other necessities are required to have a flawless distribution across the population for at least 3 years. A set time frame and a goal-oriented program are necessary to obtain observable data to study for research purposes.

For example: if there were 20 million males from puberty to 60 years of age across the country, and they were given at least one condom per week at the cost of $0.01U.S. or 0.41 PHP (Philippine currency). This is an equivalent of the staggering amount of 1.279 billion pesos for 3 years. This is just an example to extrapolate minimal data to predict future costs of condom distribution in a 3-year program (provided that this program associated with reproductive health is only limited to 3 years). This is only the cost of the condoms alone for a country, whose reproductive health care services are far from exemplary and deemed secondary to other health issues.

How about the cost of contraceptive pills, IUDs, and other devices to prevent pregnancy? Administrative services, health and legal services, educational administration and materials, jobs, and other costs to implement this program are necessary. This bill is not easily implemented throughout the country. It will create a huge monetary burden to the government within a very short period of time. The bill governing this will likely be replaced over time because of other existing prevalent problems such as crime and exploitation. Also, there is always the possibility of misuse of funds and corruption.

Meanwhile, opponents of this Reproductive Health Bill who are advocating natural family planning through abstinence practice are not really straight-forward expressing the real meaning or the whole panoramic view of abstinence. So, can natural family planning advocates just simply say to high school and college students, mature singles and married couples, that they must practice abstinence? This word is ambiguous to understand and practice for those who are poor and undereducated. This needs to be explored further. Is it something that the churches are advocating? Does one's religious faith dictate certain principles without a true understanding of the real meaning of the human body's sexual desires and abstinence?

True natural family planning is a very essential part for the growth of the nation. However, education is absolutely necessary to open everyone's eyes to see that life itself is hard enough bringing a child into this world without considering the consequences and proper preparation. The natural method is the best way to educate the whole population of teens, childbearing women, and mature men regarding pregnancy prevention versus contraceptive devices that will cost the government substantial money to implement any program.

In terms of the abstaining method as a form of natural family planning to be used as pregnancy prevention, it generally has a very shallow interpretation with the population, because it does not represent the whole idea of abstinence between a man's and a woman's sexual desire. The body's sexual sensation during intimacy is an innate part of our human existence. However, it requires a much deeper commitment and understanding to abstain naturally by knowing how to predict a woman's ovulation area of the menstrual cycle.

In this book, *Exhibit B: Prevention Guidelines* comprehensively covers all the details for men and women to prevent a woman from conceiving. This process can be used throughout one's life span and with the future offspring without any monetary funding from the government. It only requires funding for educational material to instill this practice in the school systems and with city and provincial health services to reach poor communities and rural communities in order for people to be more responsible concerning pregnancy prevention or bringing a child into this world. Instead of promoting contraceptive devices which can cause taxpayers a great deal of money to purchase, even with discounted prices, this method can save a tremendous amount of money which can instead be used for children's education and nutrition, school educational materials, school maintenance in rural villages, and other necessities for schoolchildren. It will affect not only a child's education in school, but the nature of family life.

Chapter Six

CHILDBIRTH SPACING:

Natural Form

Chapter Six

CHILDBIRTH SPACING:
Natural Form

P eople need to redefine their challenges with the facts of life. There are always tough decisions in dealing with generational differences in order to build trusting relationships. The bottom line is to get people to understand the expectations of tomorrow, where progress is waiting to correct unethical values as an excellent guideline to reinforce obligations and responsibilities.

Within the context of this idea, there is a great need to establish excellent guidelines based on ethical values to reinforce the responsibility of people regarding bringing a child, or children, into this world. The end result of this will strengthen family values and one's self-sufficiency. Otherwise, it is hard to imagine the corrosive effect of so many conflicting ideas. The easy-to-understand techniques I have introduced are commonsensical and will teach both, women and men, how to get pregnant or prevent themselves from doing so. Yet, a "no-nonsense—whatever-come-what-may" attitude always seems to be the guiding light for many couples who fail to practice proper family planning methods to bring a child into this world. These types of thoughts are true among teens as well as adults, as evidenced of multiple children in some families. People's moral values are definitely tied to their family's economics.

Childbirth spacing is an important consideration for many career women who have plans regarding how large their family size will be. They do not want to leave the size of their family up to chance. Every woman has control over this; it is not up to the man to determine that anymore. However, to do so, one must be diligent in putting to practice the principles without using unnatural, artificial, man-made contraceptive devices. The driver is the woman herself. In order to create good, acceptable childbirth spacing, women must strictly follow the guidelines set forth in *Exhibit B: Prevention Guidelines* and the men must do so also. When it's time to bring a child into this world, then, at that particular time, the couple should follow the guidelines set forth in *Exhibit A: Guidelines of Conceiving.*

Sometimes, culture, family traditions, and obligations to one's religious faith play a big role that can exert an enormous degree of persuasion to drive up public awareness about conception and pregnancy prevention. Sometimes religious faith and political motivation become roadblocks, thus, not allowing families to make the right decision for themselves and for the future growth of their families. It can also bring much stress. It is unattainable to bring a loving relationship to the next level, if people remain uneducated about the process of conception and their individual responsibilities to that process.

The only way to really re-address this issue is through education within the classrooms, as well as inner-cities' health and social services to poor and rural communities across nations. National and local government, churches, and school administrations need to promote and support all efforts toward changing people's sexual habits. There is a direct path to teach childbearing women and families the importance of a true natural family planning method and how to make smarter choices. It is an important strategy for families in making the right decisions for a better tomorrow.

Any society that is against the true natural family planning method (i.e., only using unnatural, man-made contraceptive devices) only sympathizes with the concerns of government and its problems associated with rapid population growth. Although they may aggressively endorse the unnatural, man-made contraceptive devices, it ends up being only an easy and temporary patchwork Band-Aid which obscures a permanent solution to this unending prevalent problem, and the reason is because they seek more government funding from taxpayers. Yet, the cost in money and women's health, when using these man-made contraceptive devices over a long period of time, is conveniently overlooked. Also, it can shield the true cumulative data to extrapolate observable analysis to determine a conclusive report. It is more effective to teach the true natural family planning method as set forth in this manual to educate people from puberty through adulthood and into future generations.

One objective of this book is to adapt distinctive characteristics that can be utilized to alter the sexual habits of man. It seems that old sexual habits of men die hard. People may not be readily inclined to depart from traditional methods, cultural values, as well as modern methods that are being espoused in place of cultivating ideal, natural habits. If people are willing, we can overcome bad habits and invite fresh ideas. It is important to have definite purpose and new ideas to balance a harmonious, loving relationship with each other, and allow illumination of the true meaning of the natural method to become a meaningful part of your life.

Sometimes the "Absticulate Method," the simplest and least expensive natural family planning method, may not receive much attention because bad habits have been instilled in everyone's mind for so long. Those methods are the ones being practiced time after time. However, anyone can be passionate to achieve the natural, effortless sensation of the "Absticulate Method." It can bring joy with the greatest devotion to each person as they begin to realize that this new reality is quite normal and as natural as it can be. We should, under no circumstances, take for granted the guidelines within the context of this method; instead, strive to achieve the right balance that gives a dynamic opportunity to refine those unforgettable, rewarding moments that can be enjoyed over and over again. But it all comes down to the basic natural practices with a choice of what will really work that fits with people's lifestyle.

So, in addition to the educational knowledge presented to everyone, this method decreases risks, eliminates negative thoughts, and glorifies communication among partners in child-rearing. The stresses attached to a bigger family life are removed. Our future will look brighter as we learn about the art and science of conception and pregnancy prevention in its natural form. This is the greatest gift married couples can receive.

In a normal situation when a woman menstruates regularly, the possibility of conception is always predictable as long as the man has enough strong sperm cells (not less than 48 hours old), as long as he has proper erectile of his penis, and as long as there is proper pressure to eject semen and sperm cells which can then swim up to reach and fertilize the egg cell(s), much like a heat-seeking missile that targets and hits an object no matter how many obstacles in its path.

The "Absticulate Method" is always available to do the job at any time, during any moment of intimacy. It is really an exact science if people adhere to and practice this system to create childbirth spacing in its natural form, much like cooking. It is an art and a science by itself. Like following a recipe, it takes a lot of effort to practice searching for the right ingredients to perfect the taste, one that everyone can like, and one that can inspire the imagination, exceeding expectations by remaining focused, and believing we can achieve our goal-oriented dream. We must be dedicated to overcome the existing biases and challenges associated with and expand upon natural family planning.

Today, more than ever before, people are more knowledgeable about our past as we visualize the future of our family life—a future that can shape priorities for the children of tomorrow, thereby granting us economic flexibility and educational opportunities to overcome the memories, insecurities, and uncertainties of the past. It is a beginning—a new day—to try something new.

Let's be realistic, it is not only women who are concerned about the idea of conception and pregnancy prevention. For a good family planning method, men must definitely be included in the picture and be empowered in this process. Both need to prepare their minds and bodies' natural physiological senses in order to be more effective in performing their tasks to prevent their partner from conceiving when pregnancy is not desirable. It is a true commitment to achieve one's childbirth spacing goal. The man's faithful cooperation and dedication are necessary to fulfill the family's objectives.

The purpose of a family's preplanned, oriented goal using the controlled natural family planning method is to execute an achievable, low statistical percentage of conceiving or increase a preventative percentage, as with modern contraceptives. Again, as mentioned before, the two drawbacks of these devices are: 1) health implication over the long run, and 2) financial burden to everyone who uses these products, especially the poor communities across the nation and around the world, whose access and education is limited.

Women have always been the subject of research studies about conception, pregnancy prevention, childbirth spacing, and contraceptives, despite the fact that men are actually the most crucial contributor to all these issues. It is remarkable that men's viewpoints are often absent. So, are there any such methods that exist used in privacy beside contraceptives? Everyone has the self-discipline to control their sexual hunger and/or avoid vaginal intercourse. It is a mutual agreement with and without words, an action that requires understanding to support calculated expectations. These strategies enthusiastically embrace the truthful commitment to focus on long-term intensely inspired imagination in order to maintain a long lasting loving relationship.

Furthermore, the exclusion of men by many published research papers, journals, and books on the subjects of conception, pregnancy prevention, and childbirth spacing seems to influence women to follow what has been previously written and summarized, yet, which does not represent men's perspectives. The topic of human sexuality is typically found in every issue of women's magazines in every developing country in the world today. It is time for men to acknowledge a thoughtful, courageous commitment and shoulder their responsibility regarding this subject, which will deepen trust in their relationship with their loved ones "till death do us part."

To start with, couples (new, old, or newly married) and families with multiple children should decide how many children they want or how large their family size will be, because there's no simple definitive method and criteria for childbirth spacing. It all depends on individual choices to achieve preplanned, set goals. Those who prefer the natural method need to be dedicated to the guidelines. Contraceptives should be secondary alternatives for every couple. For example, 2 years has been the standard spacing between childbirths. It means: 1 year of prevention, 3 months of trying to conceive, and 9 months of pregnancy. It really depends on what age a woman starts to bear a child and whether her menstrual cycle is normal. For example, a woman bears her first child at the age of 25, and she and her husband plan their family size to be not more than three children for the rest of her childbearing age. It is recommended for 4 to 5 years of spacing between childbirths as the appropriate goal in this situation. Therefore, by the time the third child is born, the woman is already 35 years of age.

As a women ages, her chance of conceiving decreases. So, the best way to have realistic childbirth spacing without contraceptives is to exercise a much disciplined practice, using the method here referred to as *Exhibit B: Prevention Guidelines*. Some may feel that 4 to 5 years of spacing seems too long to practice, but actually, in real time, for every month, only 10 to 12 days of menstrual ovulation area to avoid is set forth in *Exhibit B* in this book. It is the responsibility of a woman to implement a hard-nose precautionary prevention to achieve mutual preplanned goals.

Men must adhere to the prevention guidelines, especially within the critical areas of high conceiving percentage, "the ovulation area." Practice the "Absticulate Method" as much as possible. At least stay focused to uphold the guidelines of prevention without vaginal intercourse during ovulation, and take responsibility to shake off sexual desire, if necessary, to nurture a long lasting relationship and a goal that can take the relationship to the next level.

Society, which seems to oppose the true meaning of abstinence for the world beyond closed doors and instead, advocates unnatural, man-made modern contraceptives, is a hindrance to families who can practice the real natural method, like the "Absticulate Method" during the menstrual cycle, which is an option besides abstinence.

With a rapid population growth and increasing families with multiple childbirths, coupled with an increasing number of teens and other unwanted pregnancies, especially in the inner cities and poor communities across the United States and in other countries, our government health and welfare services are seriously affected, so why is this problem still lingering and cannot be contained? Even with the long lasting endorsement of modern contraceptive usage and more government funding at the expense of the taxpayers, these problems will persistently exist without the proper educational materials to educate the young and adults regarding the real and deepest sexual characteristics of men and women.

Therefore, when society finally shifts its focus on long-term growth, education will be found necessary to convey a useful and effective natural method that is healthy to every man, woman, and adolescent in the United States and around the world. The "Absticulate

Method" is always available for mankind. It is a natural method that can be practiced in a timely manner to be effective during the fertile period of the menstrual cycle. This fertile area of ovulation has always been the core topic of research studies, producing published books, many essays, research articles, educational materials, and pamphlets for health care and social services concerning conception and pregnancy prevention. And all of these promote the use of modern contraceptives.

Is it really necessary for a woman to go through any of these tortuous methods for the sake of data collection over time? The cost associated with the implementation of government's pregnancy prevention program is tremendously high—in billions of dollars—because every group that is involved in these studies and in the public healthcare services want their fair share of the pie. According to healthypeople.gov, "The average annual cost is estimated at $9.1 billion." These funds are only designated for teen pregnancies, contraceptives, and healthcare services.

A woman should have control over the method she chooses. This is an important step that gives thoughtful empowerment to women. It appears that modern contraceptive usage is designed to go hand-in-hand with the government's funded birth control program. This program is not in touch with many women's inner feelings to use a real natural method. Instead, it is part and parcel of the endorsement to use man-made modern contraceptives as a birth control method.

If this "Absticulate Method" as a genuine natural method is used as the first line of defense for the prevention of pregnancy and sexually transmitted diseases, it will not reflect cost savings right away. If implemented with the right structural composition for academic instruction, it will be the best method to educate from the grassroots level to maturity. Health and welfare, and inner-cities' healthcare services should customize and develop a program to utilize this system with families having multiple childbirths, and to prevent unwanted pregnancies and teen pregnancies, and with new arrivals of immigrants with families.

The Bureau of Education should also develop a composite of educational materials to include the "Absticulate Method" for secondary schools and college courses in human sexuality instruction. Surely within 5 years, sufficient collectible data can be obtained through the population census. If there is a tremendous drop of unwanted pregnancies, teen pregnancies, and a lower family size, then this will signify a substantial cost savings for the government's funded programs for birth control across the United States.

CONCLUSION

CONCLUSION

I n conclusion, the two methods in this book, "The Art of Conceiving and The Art of Prevention," are bigger than just what they appear to be. In truth, these methods are wider than the mind's expressive thoughts. These ideas can travel vast distances to navigate difficult, treacherous terrain everywhere to reach communities around the world, like the wind we breathe, and the ocean currents that are used as highways for sea life, crisscrossing different ocean waters around the globe, spreading everywhere. This expression gives the real meaning of "Absticulate," a method for pregnancy prevention and childbirth spacing, and the art of conceiving. It is a controlled method. It is the most basic natural practice of humans in the privacy of their bedrooms since the beginning of time. It does not involve the use of modern contraceptives for birth control. The only difference between the past and now is, of course, ancient man did not use contraceptives.

Because of technological advantages and modern man's education, it seems that we have slowly outgrown the ancient past and have become more civilized and educated, humanitarian and compassionate, and we live a more comfortable lifestyle. We can understand the natural characteristics of human beings and the overwhelming passion of man's irresistible outlook of tomorrow. We seek to reach the heavens and have a persistent, burning desire to live beyond our imagination with immeasurable skills to survive, a far cry from the tumultuous and perilous life journey of ancient man many centuries ago.

The innate sexual desire of modern man is the same as it was in the beginning of time. Their methods had no distinguishable variation to differentiate the sexual desire of ancient man of the past and modern man of the technological age of today. The only reasonable transformation of the unwritten and uncharted sexual practices of man as a natural method to be practiced is the refinement of its content into an academically modified civilized procedure that can be adequately used as a tool to educate, promote, and to curtail the sexual negligence of modern man.

This book is setting forth these ideas as guidelines for conception and pregnancy prevention in a most natural way in a passionate, comfortable atmosphere, where nature takes its course. At the same time, we keep learning new things to keep that spark alive. It is time to discuss the discrete sexual practices of man in order to educate adolescents, singles, and married people for potential growth balance, which is a precursor to overcome uncertainties and insecurities of the future and one of the determining factors for economic prosperity and a stable family life.

APPENDIX

How Eggs Develop

Eggs are female reproductive cells stored in the ovaries. Starting in puberty, **FSH** (follicle stimulating hormone) causes some of the eggs to begin maturing. Each month, one egg fully matures and is released into a fallopian tube. This process is called **ovulation**. A woman is born with her entire supply of eggs. This means the number and quality of the eggs diminish with age.

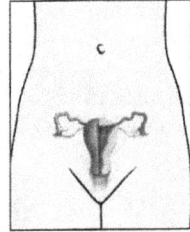

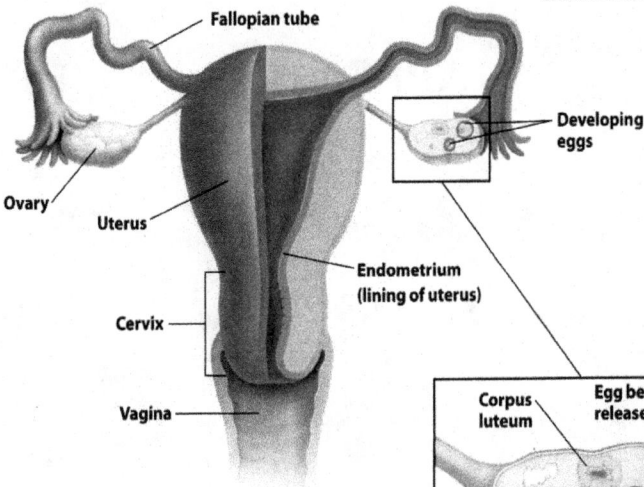

Inside the Ovaries

Each month, a certain number of eggs begin to mature within tiny sacs called **follicles**. However, only a single egg grows to full maturity. The follicles also produce **estrogen,** a hormone that thins the mucus in a woman's cervix (opening to the uterus). This makes it easier for sperm to travel through the cervix after sex.

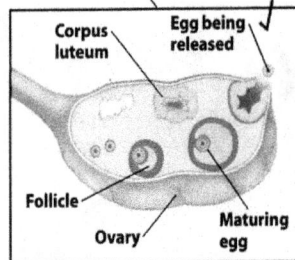

During ovulation, many egg follicles begin to develop. However, only one fully matures and releases an egg.

How an Egg Is Released

About 2 weeks after menstruation, the brain releases a chemical called **LH** (luteinizing hormone). The surge in LH causes the mature follicle to break open and release the egg. Structures on the fallopian tubes then help sweep the egg into the tube. The ruptured follicle that is left behind (called a corpus luteum) begins to release **progesterone**. This is a hormone that prepares the uterus to receive a fertilized egg.

How Sperm Develop

Sperm are male reproductive cells produced in the testicles. Starting in puberty, a man produces millions of sperm each day for the rest of his life. The production of sperm is controlled by chemical messengers called **hormones**. These are released by the brain. They include **FSH** (follicle stimulating hormone) and **LH** (luteinizing hormone). These same hormones also play a key role in female fertility.

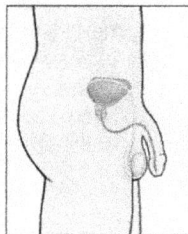

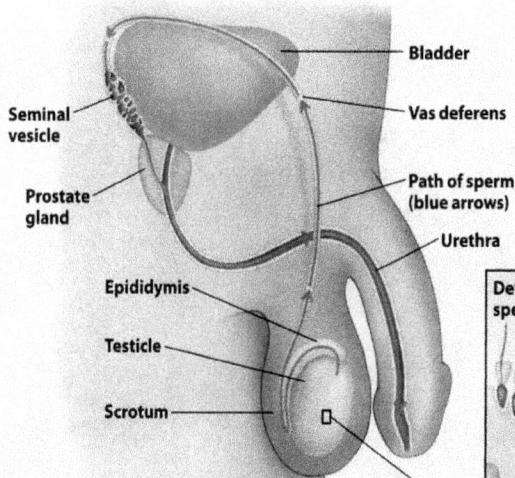

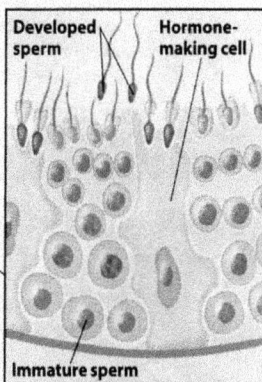

- Bladder
- Seminal vesicle
- Vas deferens
- Prostate gland
- Path of sperm (blue arrows)
- Urethra
- Epididymis
- Testicle
- Scrotum

- Developed sperm
- Hormone-making cell
- Immature sperm

Sperm developing inside the testicles take nearly 3 months to fully mature.

Inside the Testicles

FSH stimulates a man's body to make sperm. This takes place inside thin tubes in the testicles. In response to LH, nearby cells produce **testosterone**. This hormone also helps sperm develop. As the sperm mature, they move from the testicles into a coiled tube called the **epididymis**. The epididymis holds the sperm until they're ready to be ejaculated.

How Sperm Are Ejaculated

During sexual arousal, sperm are carried away from the epididymis by tubes called the **vas deferens**. Along the way, the sperm mix with fluids produced by the seminal vesicles and prostate gland to form **semen**. The semen helps nourish sperm and carry them along. During orgasm, semen is ejaculated out through the urethra.

How Sperm and Egg Meet

For pregnancy to occur, a sperm needs to fertilize an egg within 12 to 24 hours of ovulation. This is not a simple process. To reach the egg, sperm must be able to travel through the woman's reproductive tract. The fertilized egg (**embryo**) must also be able to implant in the uterus in order to grow.

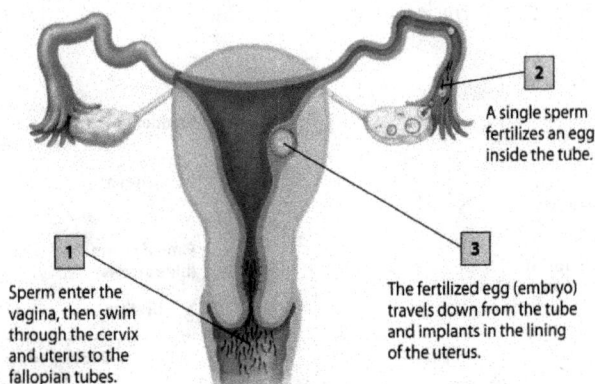

2 A single sperm fertilizes an egg inside the tube.

1 Sperm enter the vagina, then swim through the cervix and uterus to the fallopian tubes.

3 The fertilized egg (embryo) travels down from the tube and implants in the lining of the uterus.

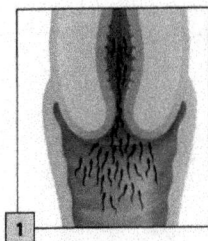

1

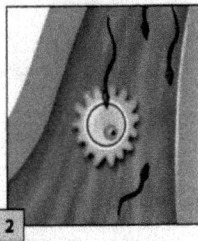

2

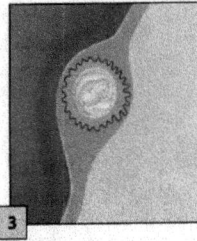

3

Sperm Enter the Cervix

After sex, sperm swim through the vagina to the cervix. There, they must be able to move through the cervical mucus in order to reach the uterus and fallopian tubes. Of the millions of sperm that are ejaculated, only a few hundred manage to reach the egg.

Fertilization Occurs

Fertilization occurs inside a fallopian tube when one sperm manages to tunnel its way through the egg's protective covering. The fertilized egg (now called an embryo) then moves from the fallopian tube into the uterus.

The Embryo Implants

About 5 to 10 days after fertilization, the embryo implants in the endometrium (inner lining of the uterus). The embryo also releases chemicals that tell a woman's body to keep producing progesterone. This helps maintain a healthy pregnancy.

REFERENCE

REFERENCES

- Ovulation: Wiegman, Stacy; Bella Online, Editor.

- Genetic Science Learning Center; University of Utah.

- *Expecting Miracles*: Zouves, Christo, MD, with Julie Sullivan: Henry Holt and Company, New York. (2003).

- Illustrations: Fertility Problems: KRAMES, Patients Education, A MediMedia, Company.

- Advanced Fertility Center of Chicago.

- healthypeople.gov

www.ingramcontent.com/pod-product-compliance
Lightning Source LLC
Chambersburg PA
CBHW070155310326
41914CB00100B/1936/J